Food for a healthy living

By

Dr.Stephanie Adams

Lawful Notification

The Distributer has strived to be just about as exact and finish as conceivable in the production of this report, despite the way that he warrants or addresses never that the items inside are precise because of the quickly changing nature of the Web.

While all endeavors have been made to confirm data gave in this distribution, the Distributer takes care of blunders, oversights, or opposite translation of the topic thus. Any apparent insults of explicit people, people groups, or associations are accidental.

In useful exhortation books, similar to whatever else throughout everyday life, there are no certifications of pay made. Perusers are advised to answer on their own judgment about their singular conditions to likewise act.

Table of contents

Introduction

In straightforward terms the body has two totally different and complex frameworks of fuel delivering sources. As energy is indispensable to the actual presence of human movement and endurance the two-energy style rely upon one another for help. This book shows you what food varieties give you the most energy.

It happens so regularly - we resolve to happen with a wellbeing and actual work out schedule with zing and probable much exhibition as well; notwithstanding, in the main seven day stretch of going into the arrangement, all that diminishes. Can any anyone explain why we don't stay with the eating regimen designs, the early daytime running plans, the actual activity designs that we make?

Also, how may we guarantee we continue onward with these plans, for the good of our own and for the people that are subject to us?

Might it be said that you are eating basically to fulfill your hunger or to make your taste buds blissful? Or on the other hand would you say you are eating to assume better control over your life? In this digital book, we perceive how you can make your life significantly more ideal basically by causing a guide that you toward eat accurately.

Chapter 1
The Rudiments

Energy is required for the different capabilities like upkeep of development, day to day exercises, practice and numerous different developments or capabilities that are frequently underestimated. These are divided among the two energy frameworks.

In this day and age, only sometimes do any wellbeing and wellness plans work. What is the justification behind their disturbing pace of disappointment? The world is much less fortifying than it was twenty years prior. Much this is ascribed to the adjusted food propensities for people.

The Nuts and bolts

The essential and first to be utilized energy framework is thc oxygen consuming framework. This framework involves oxygen for the capability of the muscles and requests a considerable amount from the general body framework.
This request normally builds the rate and profundity of breathing and blood supply chiefly in view of the comparing increment of the pulse.
At the point when the body requires more energy, which can't be met because of the raised requirement for more oxygen then the body framework consequently changed to the

anaerobic energy framework. This framework can create energy without the need to utilize oxygen.

This energy is produced through the appropriate or address utilization of food varieties. The food varieties ate direct the kinds of energy levels everybody can create. Muscle weakness ordinarily happens when all the energy sources are depleted which can be credited to different reasons; the most convincing one relies especially upon the sorts of food varieties devoured.

There are a few classes of food sources that produce different gainful components for the human body framework and taking note of the ones that make or improve the energy creating sources is helpful to be aware. Thusly, this information ought to assist the person with picking the right kinds of food sources.

The vigorous framework works by separating the sugars, unsaturated fats and amino acids in the food varieties ate while the anaerobic framework sets energy free from the food varieties put away in the body, typically during extreme movement sessions. Assuming that we catch wind of the disappointment of diets or exercise center plans surrounding us, regularly it isn't their issue.

Ordinarily the issue of the people began with much upheaval about going through these plans, leaving out nothing their associates and collaborators about it, and afterward didn't maintain those projects. The people who leave the activity or count calories midway don't see the benefits, normally, and everyone faults the arrangement.

What the world necessities these days is definitely not a new wellbeing or work out regime or an eating routine, however it requires inspiration. It needs the right kind of outlook to completely finish anything plan they have decided as far as possible.

In the event that they can do that, the greater part of the medical problems that are connected with way of life circumstances will become antiquated. Also, we don't need to visit the sides of the earth to find this inspiration. The inspiration lies here, inside us; we basically have to look through it out and use it.

One age back, people wouldn't fantasy about getting anything that unhealthy food they might set up to take care of their countenances. These days, that's what we do so nonchalantly. "I'm ravenous" regularly signifies "I need a burger or a wiener, logical with chips as an afterthought and some cola." And, "I'm on a careful nutritional plan" signifies "I'm on a synthetically ridden pill which will overcome my yearning and deny my group of nutrients." It's really no big surprise that we are confronting so many medical problems today.

Our wellbeing is a mark of what we consume. The sorry condition that we're living in is certainly not a singular issue; it's a worldwide issue. The world is eating inaccurately. Six in each ten people in the US is overweight, and the number will be eight in each ten people when we hit 2021.

Is it safe to say that we are really contemplating this? We aren't. Indeed, even as you're concentrating on this digital book, you probably have a bundle of chips as an afterthought. Do you have any idea that what you spent on that bundle, which is filling your stomach with the absolute most poisonous synthetic substances known to mankind, could rather have taken care of a thin adolescent in Ruanda?

Yet, it's not just about being humanitarian. It's about ourselves as well. Indeed, we must be narrow minded. With such shocking wellbeing figures,would we confirm or deny that we are setting out toward destruction? We're certainly not eating right. Whatever overabundance stuff that brings - stoutness and the varying medical affliction afterward - we must be ready for it.

So the following time you see that a program has fizzled or is getting a great deal of analysis, recollect that the analysis isn't likely in light of the fact that the program remains in dangerous territory. By and large, it is on the grounds that individuals started with extraordinary aims and afterward didn't follow the program as they ought to have.

Chapter 2
The Manner in which You Ponder Food

The most significant thing that you want to keep your wellbeing and work out regime alive - considerably more critical than a teacher or a specialist - is your own thought process. You not entirely settled to investigate what is going on. In this way, you're overweight and are seeing pushing off a couple of pounds.

No rec center educator from wherever on the planet will help you in the event that you don't go to sufficient lengths to have the right eating regimen and to adhere to your standard activity. Regardless of whether you're debilitated and are taking a gander at treatment, no doctor will help in the event that still up in the air in following the treatment stage, whether it's taking the prescription at the right time or going without certain food sources.

Your Attitude

We have wandered horrendously with our dietary patterns so far. Assume control over won't improve.
The number 1 thing is mindfulness. We need to realize what food varieties are right for ourselves and what are not. We need to return to preparing and fathom what the supplements are that your body genuinely needs and in what sum.

Then we need to construct a dietary routine for us as well as our friends and family with the goal that we eat better. We need to eliminate every one of the food sources that are antagonistic - the sugars, the fats, the carbs, we don't really need them - and consolidate food sources that might help our wellbeing.

This sounds excessively long winded, I get it. Yet, that is the main respite we have. Assuming we keep chomping on Oreos, we're never going to improve. Yet, there's trust. Trust lies in the way that there are a great deal of food varieties out there that are basically pretty much as scrumptious as those dreadful low quality foods yet we have hardly any familiarity with them.

These are the food sources that we have barely any familiarity with yet, we probably could do without them or as we don't have the foggiest idea how to fix them, yet a solid cookbook might help you in figuring out grouped fascinating ways to sound cooking. Indeed, even with a similar kind of diet you eat, you can invoke a few truly delectable sound dishes. Indeed, it's all a lot of conceivable. You can change your dietary patterns to a major degree, while simultaneously taking care of your sense of taste.

The truth of the matter is that the weight reduction industry is capable in a huge manner towards this defeat of the created human race.

They show us captivating before-after photos of an individual with a foot-long sub and afterward the very fellow with 6 pack abs and let us know that the eating routine made that conceivable. Nonetheless, the truth of the matter is, if we somehow managed to get our head together, we may handily do that as well, without burning through 1000s of dollars on those eating regimens. Also, what do we need to do?

2 general things: - Control what we consume. Enjoy actual effort.

Presently, is that a lot to achieve? Don't we owe that to our body that has served us so well such an extremely long time? Don't we owe that to ourselves and our friends and family?

Chapter 3

Honey And Entire Grains

Throughout the long term honey has been demonstrated to the one supporting power behind the energy circle. Helping the human body in different regions it is principal still unparalleled in its energy creating element. Honey is nature's most regular energy sponsor. It likewise goes about as a powerful insusceptibility framework manufacturer while giving the regular solution for a large group of shifted infirmities as well.

Energy is vital to the smooth streaming normal of a regular routine pattern of any individual. In this way, finding energy sources that are both steady and sound are critical to staying in shape and cheerful.

A Decent Pair

The regular advantages of honey has been generally recognized and acknowledged. Other than its incredible taste, honey is likewise a characteristic wellspring of starch, which is an energy creator for supporting execution, perseverance and lessening levels of muscle weariness.

This is particularly helpful for competitors. The sugar content in the honey assists with assuming a part in forestalling weakness during exercise meetings and furthermore during instructional courses for sports lover. These sugars make ups are partitioned into glucose and fructose and capabilities in various yet praising ways.

The glucose content in the honey is by and large consumed at a quicker rate and emits a prompt jolt of energy while the fructose works at a more slow speed for a more maintainable and drawn out energy dispensing. With regards to tending to glucose levels in the body framework, honey has been known to assist with keeping the levels steady.

As honey is a lovely food item and it's normal in its structure, devouring it's anything but an extremely challenging activity. Individuals of any age are for the most part very ready to consume honey in any of its going with structures. It's even famous with kids.

The energy delivered from consuming a modest quantity of honey day to day assists youngsters with adapting to the actual types of everyday school exercises and sports responsibilities.

For the grown-ups too consuming an everyday little portion of honey can go far in keeping the energy levels at its best during a requesting day at work. Making sandwiches with honey went with different fillings is one approach to making a wonderful bite.

Applying honey on a newly toasted cut of bread is likewise a welcome breakfast elective. Adding honey to drinks as opposed to utilizing sugar is supported. A great many people today need a convenient solution for their energy supporting necessities and this normally comes in the unfortunate types of sports beverages, espresso and refined carbs like sugar and keeping in mind that bread.

However these produce the ideal elevated energy levels, it ought to be noticed that this energy is genuinely fleeting and the sluggishness that follows is generally more intensely felt. In this way selecting to consume some type of entire grains isn't just a superior other option but at the same time is a lot better.

Entire grains give the energy that arrives in a more complicated structure what separates over a more drawn out timeframe. This then makes the stage for supporting the energy levels for longer periods.

Due to its more perplexing make up the entire grains accompany a variety of gainful components like minerals, nutrients, phytonutrients, and fiber which are additionally wealthy in fiber. Adding the entire grain fixings is any dish frequently finishes the flavor or upgrades it out and out. Entire grains can the different structures like wheat, oat, grain, maize, earthy colored rice, faro, spelt, emmer, einkorn, rye, millet, buckwheat, and some more.
These can then be made into different items like entire wheat flour, entire wheat bread, entire wheat pasta, moved oats or oat groats, triticale flour, popcorn and teff flour.

The advantages of consuming entire grains reliably can assist with diminishing the gamble of coronary illness, lower cholesterol levels safeguard against many kinds of malignant growth and aid weight the board. Entire grains ought not be mistaken for its lesser and more refined "cousin". However refined grains have a few advantages it is in every case better to decide overall grain options.

Chapter 4
Nuts And Lean Meat

Summation

Nuts are a significant wellspring of supplements for both human and creature utilization. Being wealthy in an entire host of important supplements it tends to be eaten in its crude structure, cooked or as an added substance to currently previous dishes. Thought nuts are characterized as a hard shelled natural product, there are numerous different food sources that are remembered for the nut family.

Various sorts of meats by and large add to different flavors; but the best kind is the one with however much lean meat content as could reasonably be expected. Its undisputed reality that the meats that contain a lot of fat are a culinary treat without a doubt yet for wellbeing purposes carving out opportunity to comprehend the advantages of consuming lean meats is exceptionally savvy to be sure.

Great Proteins And Oils

It is currently normal information that nuts enormously help in holding a ton of illnesses within proper limits or from happening by any stretch of the imagination.
For example, nuts have been known to have the option to keep the chance of coronary heart infections showing, in any

event, for those entire come from a long queue of relatives with this issue.

Consuming nuts like almonds and pecans have been known to bring down serum cholesterol fixations inside the body framework. Nuts are additionally enthusiastically suggested for those people experiencing insulin opposition issues like diabetics.

Going to nuts rather that unhealthy food to control desires is additionally another better other option. Containing fundamental unsaturated fats is likewise one more in addition to moment that it comes to picking nuts as a better other option. Since nuts are solid and can be consumed in its crude structure, it is likewise one more added benefit to keeping these around and convenient as tidbits.

Almonds are frequently used to standardize blood lipids due to their gradual process attributes, which help to keep the glucose levels reliably sound. Rich in a changed measure of various supplements the almond is a well known added substance to the lifeless eating regimen of most Mediterranean individuals.

The Brazil nut is likewise another nutritious nut which accompanies its own arrangement of advantages when consumed with some restraint. Noted for its omega 3 unsaturated fat substance, the Brazil nut is likewise a decent wellspring of calcium.

Cashew nut is one more exceptionally famous nut that is much of the time consumed as a salted tidbit. Anyway it would be a lot better food item without the expansion of salt, as it is now a seriously tasty nut all alone. In certain regions of the planet these nuts are made into oils.

The determination interaction ought to be finished with just enough information as relying entirely upon what the unaided eye sees isn't sufficient. For the most part lean meats got from hamburger cuts ought to incorporate round, throw, sirloin and tenderloin, while the cuts from pork or sheep would comprise tenderloin, flank hacks and leg. The most slender pieces of the poultry would be the bosom region without the skin.

However there are many reasons individuals dispense with meat from their everyday eating routine, there is no proof to show that this is a fortunate or unfortunate decision not would it be a good idea for it be trailed by all.

Anyway the significant highlight note here is the decision of the kinds of meats that would make the utilization solid and this would commonly mean meats with lesser measure of fat substance. However white meat is in no way, shape or form ailing in fat substance, it is by correlation substantially less in fat substance than red meats. The healthy benefit of consuming lean meats is very broad and adjusted.
Lean meats have a for the most part higher and cleaner content of protein which is a vital contributing element to basic primary and utilitarian advancement of each and every cell food and development.

Lean meats are likewise a decent wellspring of fundamental amino acids especially sulfur amino acids. When contrasted with the stomach related rates the proteins in meats work quicker than the one contained in the beans and entire wheat range.

Lean meat is likewise a decent wellspring of iron. Since lack of iron is moderate it is frequently not recognized until a later stage where sickliness has created.

Chapter 5
The Advantages

Here is all the thought process you'd expect to keep practicing good eating habits. How about we promptly dive into the subject.

Benefits
You GetHealthier

We could entire assortment of books about the wellbeing benefits of eating accurately yet it wouldn't exactly cover what benefits truly exist. The main benefit is that you gain control over your weight.

By eating accurately, you similarly verify that your metabolic capabilities - most strikingly your insusceptible framework and your gastrointestinal framework - continue to work accurately. You're similarly safeguarded from grouped persistent illnesses, right from cardiovascular sicknesses like coronary vein infection and hypertension to diabetes.

More Financially savvy

Practicing good eating habits implies you spend considerably less. Your bills at the grocery stores descend definitely and you don't dive farther into charge card obligation assuming that is now an issue with you. What's more, you save a colossal pack on all the medical care costs you'd require on the off chance that any issue surfaces because of your food binging habits.

Less Poisons In Your Body

A ton of food sources these days are harmful due to the manufactured synthetic compounds present in them. While you're endeavoring to eat accurately, you are significantly less prone to get these poisons into your body as one of the essential authoritative opinions of eating accurately is that you shouldn't eat anything that is man-made.

Moreover, assuming you eat less, you'll in like manner have the option to diminish on indecencies like smoking and liquor addiction. A glass of brew is practically inseparable from a night out with the young men. On the off chance that you eat less, you won't need the lager also. Likewise, you won't need that (at least one) obligatory smoke that you will more often than not have after every dinner.

More Actual Way of life

At the point when you eat better, you'll observe that you can take care of your responsibilities in a vastly improved manner. You can practice more, travel more, play more, work more and accordingly make your life more useful.

That definite beats being a fat lazy pig and relaxing around on the lounge chair the entire day, right? You can likewise be more associated with your companions and friends and family and that certainly enhances yourlife.

Great SocialLife

Disregard fat fetishism, people who are overweight don't look engaging. There's serious areas of strength for an untouchable about weight on some unacceptable spots of the body. In the event that you're attempting to find an accomplice, your fat may in a real sense disrupt the general flow. Not just that, people who have zero control over their dietary patterns and hence their weight are peered downward on by society as being people who have zero control over their basic urges.

This kind of brain science exists, however not many people will talk about it. At the point when you eat accurately, you'll find that such issues vanish.

Wrapping Up

There are a great deal of famous weight control plans available these days, however the majority of them are unfortunate and incidentally even hazardous. This will clear up how for eat a solid, adjusted diet forever and avoid unfortunate weight control plans.

Determine the number of calories your body that requires to function consistently.

This number might change fiercely, contingent upon your digestion and how genuinely dynamic you are. In the event that you're the kind of person who lays on ten hammers out plainly smelling a cut of pizza, then, at that point, your consistently caloric admission should remain roughly 2000 calories for men, and 1500 calories for ladies.

Your weight similarly has an impact in that: More calories are suitable for normally greater people, and less calories for humbler people. In the event that you're the kind of person who can eat without acquiring a pound, or you're genuinely dynamic, you could wish to build your everyday caloric admission by 1000-2000 calories, a piece less for ladies.

Try not to fear greasy food varieties.

You need to eat fat from food varieties for your body to accurately run. However, choosing the right kinds of fats: Most creature fats and a couple of vegetable oils are high in the kind of fats that raise your LDL cholesterol levels; the foul cholesterol is vital.

Unique in relation to prevalent thinking, gobbling cholesterol doesn't unavoidably raise how much cholesterol in your body. Assuming you give your body the right instruments, it will flush additional cholesterol from your body. Those instruments are monounsaturated unsaturated fats, which you should attempt to routinely consume. Food sources that are wealthy in monounsaturated unsaturated fats are olive oil, nuts, fish oil, and arranged seed oils.

Eat a lot of the right carbs.

You need to eat food sources high in carbs since they're your body's main wellspring of energy. Try to select the right carbs. Basic carbs like sugar and refined flour are immediately consumed by the body's gastrointestinal framework.

This instigates a kind of carb over-burden, and your body discharges huge measures of insulin to fight the over-burden. Not exclusively is the abundance insulin awful on your heart, but it empowers weight gain.
Eat a lot of carbs, yet consume carbs that are gradually processed by the body, for example, entire grain flour, veggies, oats, and natural grains.

Eat greater feasts almost immediately in the day.

Your digestion decelerates close to the furthest limit of the night and is less proficient at processing food sources. That implies a greater amount of the power put away in the food will be stacked away as fat and your body will not retain as numerous supplements from the feast.

Have a go at eating a medium-sized feast for breakfast, a major dinner for lunch, and a little feast for supper. Even better, endeavor consuming 4-6 little feasts over the run of your day.

Give yourself a cheat dinner.

Cheating doesn't mean glutting on every one of some unacceptable food sources one time each week; it infers partaking in a food you really love one time each week. Several cuts of pizza on Sundays, or a tremendous cut of twofold chocolate cake on Saturdays.

This cheat feast will assist you with staying with the adjustment of diet, and in a couple of ways it's truly great for your body. Exceptional events, similar to birthday events in the family, consider cheat feasts.
Get the propensity for eating gradually.

It will fulfill you with less calories and will prevent indulging and heftiness with every one of its ramifications.

Drink a lot of H2O.

It causes you to feel more conscious and stimulated, does ponders for your skin and causes you to feel more full so you end up eating less! Chopping down pop and supplanting it with water will do ponders for you.

THE END

www.ingramcontent.com/pod-product-compliance
Lightning Source LLC
LaVergne TN
LVHW041307150826
845673LV00008B/2778

9798846946033